THE ALL NATURAL

HIGH-PERFORMANCE DIET

by
Nina Anderson and Dr. Howard Peiper

Foreword by
Dr. Wm. Mundy, M.D.
author of *Curing Allergies with Visual Imagery*

Copyright© 1999 by Nina Anderson and Howard Peiper

All Rights Reserved

Edited by Arlene Murdock

No part of this book may be reproduced in any form without the written consent of the publisher

ISBN 1-884820-46-8
Library of congress Catalog Card Number 99-71261
Printed in the United States of America

The All Natural High Performance Diet is not intended as medical advice. It is written solely for informational and educational purposes. Please consult a health professional should the need for one be indicated.

Published by Safe Goods
P.O. Box 36
East Canaan, CT 06024
(860) 824-5301

FOREWORD
BY Dr. Wm. Mundy
Author of *Curing Allergies with Visual Imagery*

Our American lifestyle is the epitome of luxury. Technology has promoted material productivity, but has weakened us in many ways. Quality is sacrificed for profit, and parts are meant to wear out. When it comes to people, neither body nor brain get enough exercise. We seek to be amused, rather than creating our own pleasures through reading, conversation and relationships. The instant gratification demands of children are met with more toys and games, most of them sedentary. Encouraging creativity, making learning a pleasure rewarded with positive recognition, is too seldom a part of the modern family. Even our political system promotes rewards for no effort.

Nowhere is this trend more evident than with our eating habits. Other cultures have to eat what is available or affordable. We are able to put whatever we want on the table. To get to the TV sooner, we have microwaves to heat up shrink-wrapped, preserved foods, with so many chemical additives that we aren't sure which ones are safe or unsafe. Never mind the basic ingredients. Sadly, just as believing material goodies will make us happy, we choose foods unwisely. We are more interested in rich than lean, in the dressing rather than the salad, in cake than in bread. Emphasis is placed on healthy foods for little babies, but as soon as they are old enough to make their demands heard, we put them right on board the same nutrient-inadequate gravy train.

Once-common dietary deficiency diseases are rarely seen in America. But, how many low-level symptoms of weakness, muscle fatigue, gastrointestinal distress, headache, sexual dysfunction, memory loss and impairment of other systems might be due to nutritional deficiencies. Essential nutrients must be available not only for proper growth on a cellular level, but to maintain structure and biochemical functioning in the ever-changing milieu in which the organism exists.

For those looking to improve their health, this book may pinpoint the healing foods now missing from their diets. For those interested in taking a more active role in enhancing their physical, mental or sexual performance, this book presents a common sense approach that can easily be incorporated into today's modern lifestyle. Sometimes the very number of products known to be of benefit for any given system of the body, may seem confusing. Look at the items listed as healthy, then cater to your individual tastes and preferences and choose what works best for you.

You can feel better in every way by eating healthy foods and avoiding harmful ones. Be good to yourself. Make up your mind to help your body. Stay young longer and grow old later.

INTRODUCTION.

Have you received one of those ads in the mail about a miraculous diet pill? Do you want a sharper mind? Do you want to maintain your sexual prowess for the rest of your life—not to mention preserving your lean, mean, muscle-machine body?

Then read on. We have designed this booklet to help you make sense out of all the diet gobli-gook you hear, see and read. It is not heavy reading, and is meant to be quick reference in those times of temptation (gooey sundaes, yummy margaritas or the American standard, pizza). We give you hope towards longevity, free of decrepidation (is that a word?), senility and fat.

You are never too young to start! The earlier, the better. Teenagers are developing arthritis, aches and pains and forgetfulness. Many younger men, although they publicly won't admit it, suffer from sexual dysfunction. Athletes bulk up on steroids to replace the body's lack of performance. Sometimes, we all forget what we're saying in the middle of a sentence. The High-Performance diet can help. Even if you're over the hill, your body can do a turn around (after all, it supposedly rebuilds itself every seven years).

Of course, don't forget about exercise. It's very important. You should get a workout several times a week, especially if you're an office-chair potato. We cover only the nutrient portion of a diet, but remember, the body is a whole package. Adding mind control, exercise, relaxation and laughter make it a win-win situation.

CHAPTER OUTLINE

STEP 1... DIGESTION — 9
    FOOD COMBINING — 10
    FRIENDLY INTESTINAL CRITTERS — 14
    MUNCHKINS THAT EAT STUFF — 15

STEP 2... BALANCE BALANCE — 17
    ARE YOU ACID OR ALKALINE? — 17
    BUILDING BLOCKS OF LIFE — 19
    NO - GOO FATS — 20

STEP 3... WHAT NOT TO EAT — 23

STEP 4... MAINTENANCE — 27
    POWER PACKED ENERGY FOODS — 27
    MIND FOOD — 31
    SEX FOOD — 32
    OTHER HEAVIES FOR PERFORMANCE — 35
    AFTER THE EVENT — 40

STEP 5... THE CART BEFORE THE HORSE — 43
    JUICE FASTING AND HERBAL CLEANSES — 43
    OUR EASY FORMULA — 45
    TYPICAL MENU — 46

STEP 6... FIXES FOR PROBLEMS — 49

RESOURCE GUIDE — 53
RECOMMENDED READING — 61

So where do we start? First, throw out all your preconceived ideas of food groups, eating habits and the notion that manufacturers of the food you find in the supermarket have your best interest at heart. To make this easy, we will start at the mouth and work to the other end!

STEP 1... DIGESTION

High performance depends on your body getting nutrients from food and supplements. You can munch on organic veggies or high protein snack bars, but if they are not digested, their nutrients won't make it through the stomach wall. This means they end up at "the other end" and become very expensive toilet water.

No matter what type of food you eat, digestion starts in the mouth. You must chew your food enough times, so that your tongue can't recognize any solid pieces. Enzymes created during this process work with enzymes in the stomach and the small intestine, to facilitate the process known as digestion. If these mouth enzymes aren't mixed with the food slurry (you didn't chew enough), they won't activate enzymes throughout the food's trip to the other end. In other words, you will get very little nutritive advantage from the food you eat. Maybe the psychological high from gulping a meal is enough, but your physical body probably won't appreciate it.

Maldigestion, through what is sometimes called "a leaky gut syndrome," is a big creator of obesity and illness. Also, when the body doesn't get the vitamins and minerals it needs, we may find that the immune system is compromised. With the so-called leaky gut, food that is improperly digested may absorb into the blood stream in unhealthy forms, inconsistent with what the immune cells are used to confronting. The mind/body concept of the allergy process, recognizing that the peptide receptors on the immune cells are the same as those on the neurons of the brain (with the even more innovative possibility that the mind may actually exist on a cellular level), proposes that the immune cells, when reacting to a disease process, physical trauma or severe emotional stress, attacks these poorly digested particles as an allergen and sets up a food allergy. The particles may be completely benign in that they do not replicate nor cause infections or inflammation. Left alone, they might be taken care of by the macrophages in the blood stream, filtered out in the lymph system, or broken down as waste products and eliminated from the body through the gut or the urine. However, the immune cells, not wishing to make any mistakes in taking care of anything foreign to the body (with their assigned task against bacteria, viruses, inflammation, dead tissue, cancer, etc.), actually attacks and treats the entity as a terrorist instead of a tourist. Once the ritual of an allergy process is set up, just as the effects of vaccination are long-lasting, the allergy continues. The fewer such products that are introduced into the blood stream undigested, the less chance of a food allergy. (see Dr. Mundy's book in the reference section).

In order for digestion to take place, you must respect mother nature and eat foods in the proper combination. If you don't, the enzymes will become confused and go home. Nothing will be digested, so you will be eating just to exercise your jaw! Some food combining rules you may object to, but take heed. The choice is yours—to digest or not to digest.

FOOD COMBINING:

Yummy morsels that take the same time to digest:

2 hours:	Acid Fruit
	Melon
	Sugar (all kinds of sweeteners)
	Liquids
3 hours:	Sweet Fruit
	Dried Fruit
5 hours:	Non-starch green veggies
	Starches
12 hours:	Meat, Fowl, Fish Protein
	Fat
	Milk

The problem arises when you eat food that does not all digest at the same time. If you eat fruit and meat at the same meal, the fruit will start to ferment while it's waiting for the meat to digest. Fermentation means putrefaction which means gas, bloating and the population explosion of abnormal bacteria growth in the digestive tract. Respect this rule and watch your need for antacids disappear.

We mentioned enzymes before. There are over a thousand in the body, and they each are assigned a specific function. Those that digest meat will not digest fruit or starch and vice-versa. Therefore, to eat these foods at the same time negates any of them from being digested. When foods are not digested, you can store fat in unwanted places and inhibit muscle action.

A list of food types follows:

Non-starch Green Veggies

artichoke	garlic
asparagus	green beans
beet top	kale
bok choy	lettuce
brussel sprout	mushrooms
cabbage	onion
cauliflower	parsley
celery	peas
collard	radish
cucumber	spinach
dandelion	sprouts
eggplant	turnip
endive	zucchini

Fat

butter	oil
margarine	

Protein

red meat	fowl
fish	pork

Protein Fat
avocado
cheese & dairy
nuts
olives

soy
sour cream
yogurt (unsweetened)

Starch
beet
carrot
beans
bread
corn
grains
Hubbard squash
Jerusalem artichoke
lima bean
turnip

squash
parsnip
peanuts (raw)
potato
pumpkin
rice
seeds
soy
yam

Acid/sub-acid Fruit
apples
apricot
berries
cherries
cranberry
currant
citrus fruit

grape
kiwi
peach
pineapple
plum
strawberry
tomato

Sweet Fruit
banana
mango

papaya

Sugar
maple syrup
molasses
carob

honey
white/brown sugar
sucanat

Now for the chart. What can you eat with what?

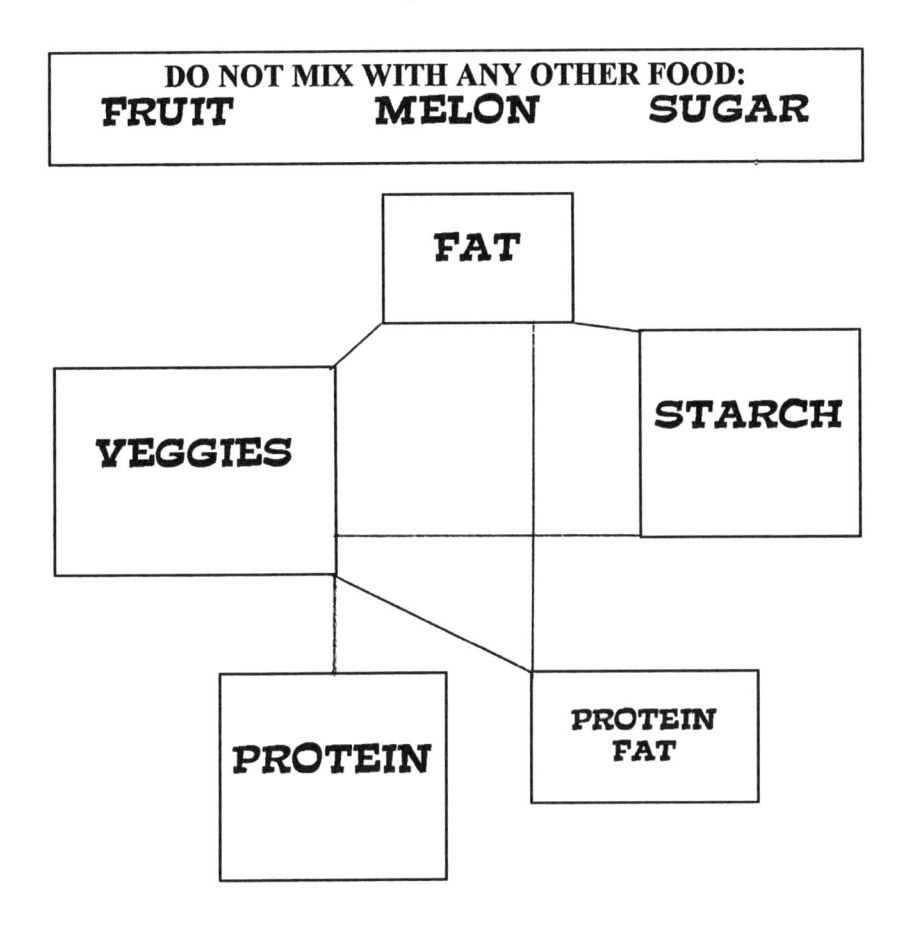

DO NOT MIX WITH ANY OTHER FOOD:
FRUIT   MELON   SUGAR

```
              ┌─────────┐
              │   FAT   │
              └─────────┘
                         ┌──────────┐
┌──────────┐             │          │
│          │             │  STARCH  │
│  VEGGIES │             │          │
│          │             └──────────┘
└──────────┘
        ┌──────────┐  ┌──────────┐
        │          │  │ PROTEIN  │
        │ PROTEIN  │  │   FAT    │
        │          │  └──────────┘
        └──────────┘
```

Changing your eating habits can be a real cultural shock. You may go into denial and defer to that roast beef sandwich or chicken and baked potato. The choice is yours. Look around at all the overweight people, and how the sale of antacids makes the manufactures rich. Many older people live out their lives hunched over and visiting doctors for aches & pains. Do you want to end up like this? Again, we say the choice is yours.

Now the clincher. You will really hate us. You can't drink with meals, and you can't drink ice-cold drinks. Diluting food in the stomach with liquid slows down the digestive process, and by drinking cold liquids it will shut down completely. So, if you want to insure maldigestion, have that cold beer with your hamburger and fries. You should drink lots of water (at least 8 glasses per day), but this should be between meals.

Another food relegated to the in-between meals status, is sugar. Dessert is an American staple, but did you know that sugar stops your digestion? That nutritious meal will now be fodder in your intestines, but you will feel happy because of that scrumptious piece of cake. If you want to indulge in sweets, do it between meals when it won't affect the rest of the food you eat.

If you do as we say—and as we do—you will start glowing internally and make your gut-brain very happy. There is such a thing, and it can be the cause of irritable bowel syndrome, among other maladies. Eating correctly, reducing stress and providing the proper bacteria for intestinal operation is the first step towards increasing your mental, physical and sexual performance.

FRIENDLY INTESTINAL CRITTERS.

As many women know, the bad guys include candida albicans, better known as yeast infections. Little known to most is the fact that these can occur throughout the body and contribute illnesses that zap our performance, such as depression, fatigue, aches, allergies, headaches, infections. Men can be affected too. Visible signs are jock-itch and toe fungus. Do you want a defense against these villains? Follow our food-combining suggestions, and then occasionally detoxify your body. Once you have killed the bad bacteria, you can rebuild the colon with friendly bacteria.

These good guys, called probiotics, come in many forms. The most common are L. acidophilus, Bifidobacterium and B. longum. Found in foods such as kefir and yogurt, these tiny warriors protect the surfaces of the intestinal mucous, produce lots of B vitamins, and fight the bad bacteria. This results in your body experience less gas, bloating, and intestinal disorders. These probiotics will complete the digestive process and help you avoid purchases of laxatives. Stomach acid can destroy these friendly bacteria when taken in supplement form. Therefore, be sure to inquire which brands are formulated to zoom through the stomach and make it to the intestines intact.

MUNCHKINS THAT EAT STUFF.

If you do what we do and do what we say, then your body will reward you with maintaining your powerful self, both inside and out. One of the key factors in digestion is enzymes that are mysterious munchkins that show up in every part of the body. They are especially useful in the intestinal tract, because they have a voracious appetite for digesting food. Without them, morsels may come out in the same form they were swallowed, and that's not good.

The pancreas makes the digestive enzymes, although it will go on strike if it works too hard. Eating cooked and processed foods requires lots of enzymes for digestion. If overworked, the pancreas gets tired—*and sick*. Also, digesting cooked foods require that metabolic enzymes, created to fight the battle against disease, must now be called in to help break down the meal. When metabolic enzymes are away from the battle ground, our immune system is more vulnerable. This leaves the body wide open for attacks from bacteria, free radicals and toxins.

If you want to do the pancreas a favor, supplement your diet with plant enzymes, every time you eat cooked or processed food. This type of enzyme works throughout the digestive tract (some just work in the stomach), and their presence will get you a thank-you note from the pancreas. Your body will love you and reward you with less stomach and intestinal diseases and even ward off arthritis, which is sometimes called the enzyme deficiency disease. It has been well-documented through animal studies, that a cooked food diet promotes a lack of enzymes in the body, resulting in old-age diseases showing up long before the animals reach old age. This applies to humans too—so pay attention!

STEP 2....BALANCE, BALANCE.

ARE YOU ACID OR ALKALINE?

Speaking of enzymes, alkaline cells are bundles of enzymes that produce energy. They create body electricity, and to be in balance, must operate in the proper acid/ alkaline range, or pH. If this balance is upset, your body could go into cellular starvation or cellular death, something which is definitely not good. Our diets have a lot to do with keeping this balance, balanced!

Since we are what we feed ourselves, when we consume primarily acid-forming foods such as sugar and meat, we are creating an environment that makes our free-radical-fighter macrophages go comatose. This gives the bad guys a free reign in our body to cause all sorts of disease and compromises in performance. If you re-balance your body with alkaline-forming foods, the macrophages will jump out of bed and go to work, keeping you healthy and strong. Don't go overboard with alkaline foods exclusively, or they will become mentally unstable and again, not perform the duties they were created to do.

Thus, you must take responsibility to maintain a balanced pH. Stress, adrenaline rushes, and other psychological events can play a part here, but at least if you control your eating habits, you'll be ahead of the game.

If you want to determine whether you are acid or alkaline, it's easy. Buy some pH-testing paper and use it with a urine sample taken when you first get up in the morning. Dip the strip in the urine and match the color with the color code on the pH paper box. Darker is more alkaline, lighter more acid. After doing this a few times, you will be able to determine which foods make your urine acid or alkaline. This will give you an indication of what you have to eat today to balance yourself. Don't forget your food-combining when making meal choices!

Alkaline-Forming Foods:

vegetables:
potato
squash
parsnips
grains
millet
buckwheat
corn
sprouted grains

beans:
soy
lima
sprouted beans

fruit:
sweet fruit

nuts:
almonds
brazil nuts
sprouted seeds

oils:
flax
olive
soy
sesame
safflower
sunflower

Acid-Forming Foods:

Protein foods:
meat
fowl
fish
pork

Beans:
lentil
navy
aduki
kidney

Fruit:
sour fruit
strawberries
cranberries

All Dairy products

Grains:
rice
barley
wheat
oats
rye

Nuts: all except above

Oils:
nut oils
butter

All Sugars

BUILDING BLOCKS OF LIFE

Next on the balance beam are minerals. Most of us are deficient in these basic elements. The glaciers do a good job of remineralizing the earth, but it's been almost 5000 years since our last fertilization. Historically, that's the time when the earth realizes its minerals have all run into the ocean and creates an ice age to replenish itself. You are drinking mineral-deficient water and eating food grown in mineral-deficient soil. Therefore, you are mineral-deficient!

What does this mean? Your structure slowly collapses. The body uses minerals as its building blocks. They make everything work right. If they're in short supply, many of the messages to the cells get short-circuited. This results in mineral-deficient symptoms such as fatigue, anemia, bone loss, senility, muscle cramps, irregular heartbeat, low sperm count and impotence in men, blood-sugar problems, obesity, gray hair, wrinkles and lots more.

If we follow all the articles in health magazines that want you to have a medicine cabinet filled with zinc pills, chromium pills, iron pills, copper pills, etc. you may be playing master-chemist with your body. This course of action will undoubtedly unbalance your body, causing more harm. The ideal solution is to take a mineral supplement that has all the needed trace minerals in the proper combination. Our favorite is a liquid crystalloid electrolyte mineral supplement. It supplies all the necessary trace minerals (there are many other minerals that your body can't use) in a form that squeezes right into the cell wall. Once inside, it helps the cell defend itself against free-radicals and other intruders, and makes it think better and work harder. Colloidal minerals are considered less effective at permeating the cell wall, because they are too big. Chelated minerals are smaller, ionic are smaller yet and have a better chance of being absorbed. Crystalloid minerals are a homeopathic form of ionic, and are so small they have the best chance of getting inside the cell wall.

If you are an athlete, you NEED minerals. Exercise, and the inevitable sweat, pour minerals out of your body. If you don't put them back in, you will age, even though your physique may look fit.

Runners many times look gaunt and experience memory loss, and women may even lose their monthly menses. This may be from lack of minerals. If you dehydrate yourself and the minerals go away, your face will sag and wrinkle. Do you want to have a dynamite body with a face that looks like a prune? Then you had better take a mineral supplement.

Speaking of dehydration, drink plenty of water. Not only is this necessary for life, but it will keep your skin from drying out. People use moisturizers to lock in water, but if you have none to lock in, what good can they do? Hydrating your body also helps remove toxins, keeps muscles pliable, provides the brain with the basis for proper neural transmissions, and helps you eliminate fat.

NO-GOO FATS.

Another balancing act comes in the form of olive oil and flax. Think about this before you eat your next fried food or salad dressing: Hydrogenated oils were created to sit on the grocery shelf without spoiling. Unfortunately, when they enter your body, they turn back into goo (trans-fats) which blocks arteries and clogs hair follicles (a key to baldness). Do you want to die so some manufacturer can put out a convenient product? Men take heed. Penile arteries are subjected to the same clogging as heart arteries. If you snack on pretzels and potato chips made with hydrogenated oil, you may be a candidate for Viagra or one of the many natural alternatives. Since a lot of our oils are hydrogenated, it's up to you to read labels.

Virgin (cold-pressed) olive oil is great. Cold-pressed means they didn't heat it during extraction, as the heating process can create carcinogens. It is high in essential fatty acids of the omega-6 variety. Most commercial oils are high in omega-6, but they need to be balanced. Omega-3 essential fatty acids are the answer. They are found in flax and fish oils. Balancing EFA's, as they are called, can prevent heart disease by thinning the blood and removing cholesterol. They also normalize the immune system, and the best part—they help to reduce wrinkles in the skin. Remember the saying, beauty starts from within? Obvious indications of EFA imbalance are brittle nails, dry skin, hair loss, depression, tinitus, cold intolerance, chronic pain, irritable-bowel syndrome, asthma, arthritis, migraines and memory loss.

Borage oil, evening primrose and black currant oils do similar good work with their GLA (gamma-linoleic acid), which acts like omega-3. The body normally creates GLA, but if you eat refined vegetable oils, have dietary deficiencies, eat sugar or have diabetes, you may require supplementation. The brain is 60% fat, and depends on dietary fat for its operation. Subscribing to a lifetime of low-fat diets, will definitely inhibit your ability to think. The amount of fat we eat is not the determining factor of health, but the quality of the fat. Essential fats are the good guys and they should never be eliminated from the diet.

Speaking of diet, there are fat blockers that can help with preventing digestion (and absorption) of fat. One of the safest is an ingredient in the spring harvested Rhododendron caucasicum plant. Found in the high mountains of the Georgian republic of the former U.S.S.R., where citizens consume this herb regularly in tea. Possibly because of the herb's strong medicinal qualities, these Georgians live to be 120 years-old. One of its ingredients has the ability to inhibit lipase (the enzyme responsible for fat breakdown). Without digestion of the fat, it is unable to pass through the intestinal wall and end up in your thighs or belly. Fortunately, essential fatty acids do not depend on an enzyme to digest them, as they are absorbed directly and are not affected by fat blockers.

A key to fat reduction comes from burning fat, instead of using up the body's principal energy carrying compound, ATP. The enzyme lipase breaks fat down into fatty acids, necessary for ATP production. Fats not broken down will cause the body to deplete ATP during exercise, causing fatigue and a slow recovery rate. If we exercise after a carbohydrate-rich meal, fatty acid release is reduced and we won't burn the fat. A low-carbohydrate food prior to exercise, helps to stimulate the release of fatty acids thereby increasing the rate of energy production (ATP). Stamina is increased and recovery time after exercise is shortened. The herb, Rhodiola rosea stimulates the release of fatty acids and makes this "food" available for ATP. During exercise these fatty acids will be converted to energy. The fat from your body will be eliminated through this process *only* if you exercise. Rhodiola rosea has been clinically proven to be extremely effective in weight loss programs.

Now comes the startling evidence. What is not food, that comes in your food, but is really a chemical that can harm your body? Several items are BHT/BHA, Ethoxyquin, Artificial color, Propylene Glycol, Sodium Nitrate and Sodium Nitrite, EDTA, MSG, Aspartame, Polyvinyl chloride, Styrene. *Here are the No-No's*.

STEP 3....WHAT NOT TO EAT.

We'll give you a little run down on the things manufacturers do to your food to make it look prettier, taste better, last longer on the shelves and save them money. Do they really consider your health? Maybe so, maybe not. But, why be the guinea pig? Here are a few of the culprits. You make your own decision.

ARTIFICIAL COLOR. Most people are aware of the toxic side effects of artificial colors and flavors from coal tar derivatives such as Red #40, a possible carcinogen, and Yellow #6, which causes sensitivity to viruses and has caused death to animals. Cochineal extract or Carmine Dye is a color additive used in food, drinks, cosmetics and to dye fibers red. It is made from the ground up female cochineal bugs from Central and South America. University of Michigan allergist, James Baldwin, M.D., confirmed cochineal extract triggered life-threatening anaphylactic shock in some people.

ASPARTAME. This very popular sugar substitute, known as Nutrasweet, has very adverse effects on the human body. It contains Methyl Alcohol, a highly toxic poison that can cause recurrent headaches, mental aberrations, seizures, suicidal tendencies, behavioral disorders, birth defects, skin lesions and urinary bladder disturbances. The Nutrasweet "hangover" may consist of malaise, nausea, headaches, dizziness, visual disturbances and convulsions. It has been implicated in Parkinson's disease and as a contributor to Alzheimer's. For more information, read Dr. Russell Blaylock's book, *Excitotoxins: The Taste that Kills*.

BHT/BHA. Used to stabilize fats in foods, these petroleum products have caused reduced growth rate in animal studies. Human reactions to BHA are skin blisters, infertility, liver and kidney damage, hemorrhaging of the eye, weakness, and discomfort in breathing. The International Agency for Research on cancer, considers BHA to be possibly carcinogenic to humans, and the State of California has listed BHA as a carcinogen. Some studies show the same cancer causing possibilities for BHT.

EDTA. This substance is used to prevent fat and oil products from going rancid, and also keeps fruits and veggies from turning brown. When present in excess, it can cause kidney damage, calcium imbalance, and mimics symptoms similar to certain vitamin deficiencies.

ETHOXYQUIN. Originally designed as a rubber stabilizer and herbicide, it is used as a preservative. It has contributed to liver/kidney damage, cancerous skin lesions, loss of hair, blindness, leukemia, fetal abnormalities and chronic diarrhea in people who work with this chemical.

MSG. Most people are aware of the dangers of MSG and request it be withheld from restaurant foods. MSG, an excitotoxin, has been found to damage the retina of infant rats, and destroy nerve cells of the hypothalamus. Humans exhibit headaches, tightness in the chest and burning sensations in the extremities. Dr. John Olney of the Washington University School of Medicine in St. Louis, MO, notes that children are more susceptible than adults to the effects of MSG. Adults have well-developed blood brain barriers that act as protectors from toxins. Children's brains are less fully developed. Therefore, with less protection, damage done to the brains of young children can be permanent.

OLESTRA. This is a new fake fat, recently approved by the FDA. It is made from refined cottonseed oil and soybean oil from which glycerin is removed and regular table sugar is added with the help of a catalyst. Since our digestive enzymes cannot break down the resultant sucrose polyester molecules, the olestra passes through the body undigested. This can cause gastrointestinal problems. In addition, this additive attaches to valuable nutrients (like beneficial cartenoids), and flushes them out of the body leaving us less protected from toxins. Found in breads, pastries, candy, snack food and Olestra™, it is a potent allergen that can trigger anaphylactic reactions in people who have asthma or allergies. The Harvard School of Public Health states that "the long-term consumption of olestra snack foods might result in several thousand unnecessary deaths per year as well as causing diarrhea and other serious gastrointestinal problems." Even the label warns us against use: *Olestra may cause abdominal cramping and loose stools. Olestra inhibits the absorption of Vitamins A,D,E, and K and other nutrients.*

PESTICIDES. To maintain a healthy diet you must avoid pesticides. Found just about everywhere, pesticides are altering our genetic makeup, producing animal and bird mutations, and insuring eventual demise of the planet. Most obvious is the assault to health, manifesting itself as cancer. Pesticides are implicated in the loss of sexual libido of both sexes. This is due to the fact that they mimic estrogen when absorbed into the body and upset the normal hormonal balance. Fruits and vegetables that are most susceptible to contamination from pesticides (unless you choose organic varieties), in order of highest risk of contamination are: strawberries, bell, green and red peppers, spinach, cherries, peaches, cantaloupe (from Mexico), celery, apples, apricots, green beans, grapes, cucumbers.

PROPYLENE GLYCOL. Used as a de-icing fluid for airplanes, this chemical is added to food and skin products to maintain texture and moisture as well as inhibiting bacteria growth in the product. It also inhibits the growth of the friendly bacteria in your intestines and decreases the amount of moisture in the intestinal tract leading to constipation and cancer.

SODIUM NITRITE. Used in the curing of meats, this substance participates in a chemical reaction through heating (cooking) that becomes carcinogenic.

THI (a browning agent). An immunosuppressant/Carcinogen, cola drinks and processed brownish foods, get their color from an ammonia caramel compound called THI. The patent for THI is for its immune suppressing qualities. Foods and drinks containing THI may look better, but by suppressing your immune system, can open the door for illness.

UNFERMENTED SOY. Unfermented soy products (tofu, soy milk, soy cheese, etc.) contain enzyme inhibitors that prohibit soy from being digested. This leads to an overworked pancreas and deficiencies in amino acid uptake. It is also high in phytates which block assimilation of essential minerals in the intestinal tract. If meat is eaten with soy, this effect is reduced. Fermented or sprouted soy has lost its enzyme inhibitors, and therefore will allow digestion and absorption to take place. This form of soy can provide all the nutritious benefits of this bean, without the hazards.

If you follow our recommendations, you will give your immune system a real shot in the arm. It will begin doing the things it's supposed to do. You will find that you'll have more physical and sexual stamina, a better memory, fewer colds, less indigestion, more energy. Your skin will exhibit a healthy, smooth and wrinkle resistant appearance. Remember, your outsides reflect the state of your insides.

STEP 4....MAINTENANCE.

POWER PACKED ENERGY FOODS

When carbohydrates are available, protein is not used for energy. When these carbohydrates are not available, the body converts protein into glucose. Protein is also used when low oxygen levels block the use of fat for energy. Protein plays an essential role in the production of hormones and new muscle tissue. To maintain existing cells, one must replace lost protein, and to build new tissue, we must consume more protein than was lost. The RDA for protein is 60mg. per day for adults, although requirements rise with strenuous exercise. When athletes need to improve performance and stamina, they increase their protein. If intake is inadequate, the body takes the needed proteins from lean tissue, as seen in many marathon runners' gaunt appearance.

Any vegetarian will tell you the importance of green vegetables. Any meat eater will tell vegetarians they're not getting enough protein. Free-range animal sources are a good source of protein, but plants are even better! Wheat and barley grass extracts (juice or powder) actually contain 25% protein whereas milk is 3%, eggs 12%, and steak is 16%. So, if you're worried about protein, take these powdered dehydrated cereal grasses every day and worry no more! They also contain anti-cancer agents, such as vitamins E and A, Zinc and the trace mineral selenium, thereby helping to promote longevity. Wheat and barley grasses also have lots of vitamin C and bioflavonoids that can slow down cellular oxidation, a fancy name for cellular aging.

Another non-meat source of protein is whey. Many companies add whey to their sports powders, but not all whey is alike. Whey is naturally high in lactose (a milk sugar that is hard for some folks to digest) and fat. Scientists have developed a method to remove the lactose and fat from the whey protein and give us a healthier product. They also change molecular structure to provide a more bioavailable substance. Properly processed whey protein is ideal because is lactose free, low in calories, and contains near zero carbohydrates. It is predigested for maximum absorption and provides a form of amino acids that is easily converted into glucose for energy.

Another green food, found in several supplements, is also an anti-aging food. Chlorella, a single cell algae, doesn't know how to die and teaches your cells how to resist becoming decrepit. Human RNA/DNA production slows down as people age, which is one of the causes of disease and lower energy levels. Eating foods rich in RNA/DNA, such as Chlorella, shores up our cell walls and helps to repair our own genetic material, thus helping to reverse the aging process. Chlorella also stimulates the macrophages (free radical eliminators), thereby protecting you from bacteria, viruses and cancer cells.

Chlorophyll, called "concentrated sun power," is the blood of the plant and is very effective against bacteria which can gain a foothold if your immune system is down. It can actually be more effective than vitamin A, C or E as an antioxidant. It also helps to alkalize blood pH. Chlorophyll, in some cases, acts to support the adrenal glands in women who are experiencing menopause symptoms. When adrenal gland function is reduced, it can compound low estrogen conditions such as hot flashes, mood swings and headaches. Chlorophyll can act as a weak replacement for estrogen, thereby boosting adrenal function. Environmental factors can cause cellular mutation (change DNA) which accelerates aging. Chlorophyll helps to nullify those environmental invaders.

Sea vegetables such as kelp, spirulina and other algae, provide a high source of micronutrients that can help decrease symptoms of PMS and cystic breast disease. They improve the condition of hair, assist in re-growth (a plus for balding or thinning mops) and also have been known to bring color back to gray hair. Kelp sparks vital enzyme reactions in the body and increases thyroid metabolism therefore it becomes effective in weight control. It also has been shown to lower blood pressure and cholesterol, two factors which definitely can lead to a longer life.

Carbohydrates are a relatively poor source of long term energy. Fatty acids are the richest source of energy production in the body. Flax bars can provide an excellent energy boost. High in essential fatty acids, flax is like oiling the inside of your body. Increased fatty acids mean increased flexibility, especially in the most active tissues such as the brain and eye. Unsaturated fatty acids also attract oxygen and aid in its transport to needed areas throughout the body. As a complete protein, flax helps build muscles, blood, internal organs, skin, hair, heart and the brain. It has complex carbohydrates that give us instant calories for energy, as well as regulating our fat metabolism. Because of its high fiber, it reduces hunger pangs. Instead of a quick chocolate bar before your next performance endurance event, try a flax energy bar. You'll get twice the energy with none of the sugar-induced side effects of fatigue, lightheadedness and hunger, which usually appear several hours later (when the sugar wears off).

In addition to food, many athletes gulp down power drinks before an event. Unfortunately, many of these contain ingredients that do not have energy-sustaining values. Most contain sugar, which can give you a burst of energy, only to drop the bottom out of your stamina an hour later. Mineralized water is far better. The electrolytes cause your brain to spark, and when your brain is running optimally, the rest of your body also gets the message. There are sports drinks available that not only contain electrolytes, but antioxidants as well. This is extremely important, as performance depends on a strong immune system.

One of the strongest antioxidants is garlic, known as a natural remedy for centuries. It's been called the miracle cure, used for colds, sore throats, topically to ward off wound infections, and as protection from virus, bacteria, parasites and fungus. But, the downside is garlic breath. Leave it to science to come up with odorless garlic supplements (aged garlic extract) which actually are more beneficial than raw garlic in many instances. Much research into the benefits of aged garlic extract (AGE) has been done, and we now know how truly beneficial this little clove is.

AGE studies have shown it lowers serum cholesterol by interfering with its synthesis in the body. Memory improves in Alzheimer's patients and it also enhances brain nutrition. AGE offers liver protection, prevents cancer, reduces blood clot formation (when it's not needed for wound healing), inhibits Candida albicans (the bad intestinal bacteria) and helps strengthen the good colon flora. It keeps blood from sticking to arterial walls, thus preventing arteriosclerosis, and acts as an effective free-radical fighter.

AGE is very helpful at stress reduction by lowering corticoid, a hormone secreted by the body during performance stress. AGE and its constituents S-allyl cysteine, allixin and diallyl sulfide have been shown to inhibit breast cancer, bladder cancer, melanoma cells, skin, liver, lung and colon cancer. It can prevent hair loss, fight ear infections, relieve arthritis pain and bouts of colitis, zap athlete's foot and help diabetics. I could go on, but I think by now you have gotten the point and will be afraid not to add garlic or better yet, aged garlic extract to your diet.

Another strong antioxidant is polyphenol, found in plants such as the Rhododendron caucasicum. Most of us have heard of proanthocyanidins, found in grape seed and pine bark. These types of antioxidants were thought to be responsible for the curing effects of grape seed. Remember when we talked about minerals and said colloidal was a form too big to be absorbed into the cell? Well, proanthocyanidins are too big, and although they are effective at helping cardiovascular conditions, since they are not absorbed into the cell, their antioxidant properties are minimal. The smaller, more absorbable form of antioxidant is a polyphenol, and when extracted from the grape seed or Rhododendron caucasicum plant, can provide a superior antioxidant for the body.

MIND FOOD.

A neurotransmitter is the chemical language sent between cells in the human brain. These neurotransmitters allow the brain cells to talk to each other. Deficiency in neurotransmitter function results in depression, lifelessness, moods, irritability, sleeplessness, anxiety, brain fog, cravings and addictions. Depleted supplies of the "feel good" neurotransmitters make it difficult for you to feel happy, on track and motivated. Neurotransmitter deficiencies can be caused through genetics, stress, diets low in amino acids, and through alcohol or drug abuse.

Two key amino acids are necessary to make the other neurotransmitters. Phenylalanine is an essential amino acid that makes you feel happy and motivated. Glutamine is a conditionally essential amino acid that can keep you calm, focused and in control. (Please note that the natural food supplement Phenylalanine should not be confused with the chemically altered form of phenylalanine which is in the artificial sweetener, aspartame.) In order to function properly, the body must have the essential amino acid, Phenylalanine. Since the body cannot convert this from other nutrients, it must depend on outside sources and specific supplements to acquire sufficient amounts. Since amino acids from meat, eggs and dairy sources cannot readily be utilized by the brain, it is necessary to take supplements which also contain co-factors that help them cross the blood-brain barrier.

The Rhodiola rosea extract has been shown to influence learning and memory, by supporting neurotransmitters and affecting brain chemistry. Tests using Rhodiola showed the quality of the task performed was dependent on fatigue levels. When Rhodiola was administered, it effectively increased a person's resistance to fatigue, enhanced back muscle strength, hand-strength endurance and improved coordination.

Neurotransmitter support is necessary for the brain to function at top performance. Memory loss may be nothing more than an amino acid deficiency, causing a short circuit. When athletes compete, they adequate brain activity to keep focused. Poor diets and low amino acid levels will prevent this. No matter what we do, our thinking process determines the outcome of our actions. With good neurotransmitter support we can make choices that can keep us at peak performance.

SEX FOOD.

Minerals, "good" fats, and amino acids can help increase sexual performance. A high-fat diet will actually decrease sexuality. Men who eat a high-fat meal will have an immediate 25% drop in their testosterone levels and women will tend to feel sleepy. Improper balance of fats may create a high level of LDL cholesterol that reduces the ability of the penis to receive 'erection signals' from the brain. When the arteries are clogged due to a high-fat diet, penis tissue flexibility is reduced, which results in the shortening and weakening of erections. Eating a low fat diet may help, but remember what we previously said about compromising the essential fatty acid levels in your body?

If the brain is fat deficient, proper signals will not be sent to the sexual organs and performance will be compromised. Essential fatty acids (EFAs) help provide moisture and softness to the skin, bladder, and in women, the vagina (especially important when estrogen level decreases). Essential fatty acids increase energy levels, especially physical activity. We tire less quickly, recover faster, feel more like being sexually active, and stay alert later in the evening. An excellent source of EFA's is Flax seed (also known as horny food).

Minerals play a big part in keeping us sexually fit. In men, one of the main physical causes of impotence is atherosclerosis of the penile arteries, which restricts blood flow. This can be traced back to mineral imbalance. It is thought that in a significant number of men, hardening of the arteries is caused by a diet too high in certain fats and sugars. What is not considered is that this problem may be caused by a lack of trace minerals, including chromium and manganese. Chromium can also reduce mood swings that contribute to loss of libido, whereas manganese is involved in female sex hormone production.

Another mineral, calcium, when taken with magnesium, acts as a natural relaxant to assist in treating performance anxiety. Magnesium contributes to the production of sex hormones. This mineral is also beneficial for counteracting depression. Phosphorus is essential to support brain and nerve activity. When taken with calcium and magnesium, it helps maintain sexual desire. Phosphorus increases muscle performance, while decreasing muscle fatigue—important for stamina in men. Selenium is needed for sperm production. It also helps women promote progesterone. Zinc is of major importance in the male reproductive system. One of zinc's many roles is in the stimulation of the male hormone, testosterone. This hormone assists in men's capacity to develop an erection, and to ejaculate. Infertility and loss of sex drive may be the result of a zinc deficiency.

Certain amino acids (protein) have proven to be important for men addressing infertility problems. L-Arginine may help increase sperm production and motility, besides being the well-known boost for the hormone testosterone. Tyrosine boosts dopamine levels (associated with memory ability, sense of well-being and with sex drive). Phenylalanine is one of the essential amino acids that is a neurotransmitter precursor influential in sexual arousal and response. Nutritional yeast is an excellent source of protein that contains Vitamin B complex and amino acids.

New sexual performance elixirs on the market include Rhodiola rosea and velvet antler. When harvested (by a method that doesn't hurt the elk/deer) at a certain time of the year, velvet antler becomes a very potent source of hormones, minerals, amino acids and enzymes. Chinese doctors have used antler velvet for male incontinence, prostatic problems, and enlarged prostates for thousands of years. For women, besides helping with frigidity and infertility, the antlers contain a high amount of calcium, useful in preventing osteoporosis. Rhodiola rosea has been known as a powerful stimulant for centuries. In studies, this herb was found to help patients suffering from weak erection, premature ejaculation, poor sleep, irritability and sweatiness.

Horny Goat Weed is a stimulating herb with androgenic-like effects that lowers blood pressure by vasodilation. This herb stimulates hormone release, is a powerful sexual stimulant and has been used in Chinese medicine for various conditions of sexual dysfunction. Mucuna Pruriens is a potent Ayurvedic herb that is the best source of L-dopa (a substance that crosses the blood-brain barrier, converting to Dopamine). In the brain, Dopamine is a very powerful neurotransmitter that regulates sex drive, resulting in heightening libido and increasing sexual performance. Maca, a root herb from Peru, is used for infertility, menopause, libido, hormonal irregularities in men and women including PMS and menstrual problems. Camu-camu, also from Peru contains powerful phytochemicals that help with depression, mental acuity, and headaches. Muira Puama or potency wood, has been traditionally used in the Brazilian culture for sexual support and to reduce frigidity. Tribulus Terrestris, mostly found in India and Africa, has been used to treat infertility, impotence and loss of libido.

Wheatgrass is an excellent source of protein and essential fatty acids. Viktoras Kulvinskas in his book, *The Lover's Diet*, says that wheatgrass is the highest vibrational food on the planet. People who eat wheatgrass have reported an increase in stamina. Lecithin, a fat-like substance normally produced in the liver, is another food supplement that aids sexual performance. Combining lecithin and crystalloid electrolytes will slowly rebalance and eliminate the problem of penile dysfunction. Lecithin is an important constituent of both vaginal and seminal fluids. It also affects the sex center of the brain, the transmission of nerve messages for sexuality, and the endocrine glands

Human Growth Hormone (HGH) is the latest addition to the longevity marketplace. Replacing what mother nature loses as we age, growth hormone offers a wide variety of health benefits. Our body produces less growth hormone as we age causing imbalances in our hormonal levels of estrogen, progesterone, testosterone and melatonin. Supplementing with HGH can help restore this balance. The benefits of growth hormone supplementation can be on or any of the following: improved stamina, sounder sleep, increase in energy, improved muscle tone, weight loss, enhanced sexual function, increase in strength, improved mental process and emotional stability. Natural progesterone has been recommended by alternative medicine physicians for twenty years. The medical community is now finally recognizing that estrogen dominance is creating imbalances in the body reducing progesterone levels resulting in lack of sexual libido.

When we eat pesticide-laden food or breathe air filled with environmental chemicals, we are putting xenobiotics into our bodies. Xenobiotics are substances than look like estrogen to the body and can unbalance our hormones. The animal kingdom is influenced by xenobiotics. Various species exhibit symptoms such as birds laying soft eggs, infertile species, birds that won't mate, alligators with undescended testes, deformed offspring and diseases like cancer that don't show up until later in life. We can protect ourselves by eating organic and avoiding chemical products. Since most of us have already been exposed, we may actually be hormone-imbalanced. By adding a natural progesterone creme supplement to our daily regime, both men and women may rebalance their bodies and restore sexual energy.

Subtle organizing energy fields (SOEFs) improve cell function. Nutrients are defined as that which energizes the SOEFs: sunlight, oxygen, live organic foods and tachyon energy. Tachyon is a theoretical subatomic particle that moves faster than the speed of light with real energy, but no mass. It is known as the life force energy. When it is blocked, our electrical system can short circuit and prevent healing. By using SOEFs including Tachyonized products, we can clear such blocks. For the first time in history, we have scientific methods of restructuring certain materials at the sub-molecular level, that then become antennae to attract and focus usable biological energy, i.e., Tachyon energy.

OTHER HEAVIES FOR PERFORMANCE.

BEE POLLEN. This is the bee's vitamin pill as it contains vitamins, minerals, enzymes, amino acids, lecithin and fructose. It's used to treat anemia, obesity, diarrhea, skin problems and mental illness.

BIOFLAVONOIDS. Referred to by some as vitamin P, bioflavonoids are the largest group of antioxidants that fight free radicals (the bad guys), which cause cellular damage. They also help alleviate the symptoms of asthma, assist in lowering cholesterol, enhance capillary and vein strength to reduce male sexual dysfunction, protect connective tissue, and reduce bruising.

CALCIUM/MAGNESIUM. These two minerals should never be separated. There is a lot of hype on taking calcium supplementation to prevent osteoporosis, but rarely is magnesium mentioned. The latter is a carrier for the former, therefore without magnesium, calcium won't make it to the bones. Silica also influences uptake of calcium. Taking too much calcium alone actually depletes the body of magnesium and makes the calcium itself unabsorbable. Too much calcium can also disrupt the body's levels of zinc, iron and manganese. So, it's important if you supplement your diet, take calcium and magnesium in a 1:1 ratio. If you take diuretics, you must add back the calcium, magnesium and potassium that is excreted.

CHROMIUM. As an aid to glucose metabolism, chromium is essential to the regulation of blood sugar. It protects against cardiovascular disease, diabetes, high cholesterol, and helps to decrease body weight. Supplementation is essential if you eat white flour, milk and sugar, as those foods steal chromium from the body and excrete it unused. Nutritionally speaking, chromium is not well absorbed. As a result, a chelating agent or picolinate, needs to be combined with chromium, which allows it to bond with the other trace minerals.

FLOWER REMEDIES. Homeopathic extracts from specific flowers principally treat the personality state (mental and emotional) of a person. Many flowers will directly influence physical symptoms and disorders. Each flower has a distinct signature (smell, color, shape, location of growth), defining its particular therapeutic value. Flower combinations have the power to balance and change energy patterns in the human bio-electromagnetic energy field affecting mood, attitude and performance. Flower remedies are listed as to the malady you are trying to correct. They can be taken internally or applied topically.

HERBS. Specific herbs are useful for increasing performance. Gingko biloba is an important herb for strength, vitality, mental alertness, and to enhance vitality levels. Ginseng is the best known of the so-called aphrodisiac herbs. Kava kava and ginger work together to produce a mild euphoria, and act as a relaxant. Maca, a Peruvian herb, promotes mental clarity, increases energy and gives athletes' stamina. Camu-camu is effective against headaches and anxiety. Saw Palmetto is a natural steroid used to increase libido, and as a mild aphrodisiac in women. Rhodiola rosea is effective for treating memory, Parkinson's and as an aphrodisiac. Rhododendron caucasicum helps allergies, arthritis, various heart problems and is a powerful antioxidant.

IRON. For people who exercise less than four hours per week, iron deficiency is as much concern as for a sedentary individual. For athletes working out more than six hours per week, their use of iron stores could bring on anemia. Especially important for teens who engage in many sports activities, iron replenishment may be a necessity (10 to 15 mg./day from food or supplements). If anemia is not suspected, refrain from adding iron, as overdoses raise the risk of heart disease and colon cancer. In cases of sexual dysfunction, iron may be used to nourish an under-active thyroid, which affects the rate at which sex hormones are created.

LECITHIN. This fat-like substance is normally produced in the liver if the diet is adequate. Nutrients enter and leave your cells via cell membranes mostly composed of lecithin. If it's in short supply, this membrane will harden and nutrients will be kept out. The best thing lecithin does is to dissolve the bad cholesterol in the blood. It can also help with memory loss, assist with absorption of fat soluble vitamins because it's an emulsifier (makes two unlike substances able to merge), relieve angina and lower atherosclerosis.

NUTRITIONAL YEAST. This nutrient is great to give to your pooch or kitty as a flea preventative, but it is also good for their owners. It is a concentrated source of B vitamins and minerals (iron, potassium, calcium, chromium) and is a high quality protein with very little fat. The chromium is chemically linked to niacin and amino acids, in order to increase the effectiveness of the body's own insulin that regulates blood sugar. It therefore is very important for fighting diabetes and cholesterol-induced heart disease.

NATURAL PROGESTERONE. This hormone, produced both in men and women, can be the key to many performance difficulties. It is the basis for the production of other hormones including testosterone. A reduction in the body's natural progesterone can create an over-estrogen condition. This results in lack of libido, PMS symptoms, migraines, prostate problems, infertility, and menopausal problems. Pesticides and other chemicals in the environment can mimic estrogen in the body, and contribute to the imbalance. Natural progesterone from the processed wild yam is best taken in cream form where it can be absorbed directly into the body.

RHODIOLA ROSEA. This herb, a Russian secret for centuries, has active ingredients that are effective against heart disease, depression, cancer and stress. It is used to enhance mental and physical performance, and to strengthen the immune system. Rhodiola rosea enhances performance by decreasing the level of exertion of the regulatory system under physical stress. This helps the body to compensate for the stress of exercise, and re-route necessary nutrients to the muscles, heart and lungs. Rhodiola also enhances a person's ability for memorization and prolonged concentration. In a proofreading test, those taking the extract decreased the number of mistakes by 88%.

SELENIUM. In many areas of the country, this mineral is in short supply in the soil. Therefore, it may not be present in the food we grow. Selenium is a free-radical scavenger, assisting in removing toxins from the body. Deficiencies can cause cellular damage from prolonged exercise, resulting in muscle fatigue. If supplements are taken with vitamins A and E, it has been reported to help against breast tumors by promoting release of progesterone. Any supplementation should be done sparingly as only trace amounts are needed to be effective. Also beware of taking lots of vitamin A as overdoses have reported symptoms of deep bone pain, headaches, hair loss, and dry skin.

SODIUM. This element helps cells retain water and prevents dehydration. It also helps generate ATP (your body's energy maker). If exercising for long periods in hot weather, beware of sodium depletion through sweat. Eating salt is not the answer, as the sodium in salt may not be bioavailable (absorbed) to the cells. Sodium supplementation is a better choice.

VELVET ANTLER. When harvested (by a method that doesn't hurt the elk/deer) at a certain time of the year, velvet antler becomes a very potent source of hormones, minerals, amino acids and enzymes as well as cartilage. Elk and deer in their natural setting eat a variety of herbs, including ginseng, which is considered an aphrodisiac. Velvet antlers contain both the male and female hormone precursors. One of the hormones, testosterone, is extremely important in that it stimulates growth, sexual potency and desire in both men and women. Chinese doctors have used antler velvet for male incontinence, prostatic problems, and enlarged prostates for thousands of years. This may be attributed to other parts of the antler such as the anti-inflammatory prostaglandins and the anti-inflammatory portions of the cartilage. For women, besides helping with frigidity and infertility, the antlers contain a high amount of calcium, useful in preventing osteoporosis. It may also help in the treatment of menstrual disorders.

VITAMIN E: An excellent antioxidant, vitamin E prevents cellular damage during exercise. Aerobic exercise places additional demands on the free-radical scavengers of the body, such as vitamin E. Therefore, replacement of these lost "good guys" is essential. A daily dosage of 800 IU can significantly decrease oxidative damage to muscle tissue.

ZINC: This mineral aids in post-exertion tissue repair through the conversion of food to fuel. Studies correlate endurance exercise with periods of compromised immunity, possibly because of zinc depletion. Constant aerobic training may accelerate zinc loss, and thereby put the athletes' immune system at risk. Zinc deficiencies can cause an imbalance in copper levels. When these are too high, they can contribute to hyperactivity and confused brain function, such as symptoms found in children with A.D.D. Supplementing with 30 to 60 mg. per day, can replace depleted stores.

Men will love zinc (along with the herb Saw Palmetto), as it helps with prostate problems This mineral has a long list of reasons to take it. Zinc can reduce inflammation, tone down body odor, boost the immune system, prevent toxic effects of heavy metals like cadmium, improve fertility and sexual potency. It can also help reduce night blindness and reduce swelling and stiffness for arthritis sufferers. However, beware of playing master chemist as overdoses can lead to fever, nausea, vomiting, diarrhea, and cause iron and copper to leach from the body, contributing to anemia.

AFTER THE EVENT.

It is important to put back nutrients that are used up due to exercise, stress or mental strain. Water is the number one replacement item. Rehydration is extremely important to facilitate restoration of muscle tone and bodily function. Exercise can make us lose the equivalent 1 ½ gallons of water through sweat. Marathon runners metabolize about ¾ pound of fat, but lose up to ten pounds of water weight. Drinking water with added electrolytes is the best choice. Electrolytes facilitate the removal of lactic acid build-up in the muscles, which contributes to the soreness and stiffness we feel the day after our workout. Some drinks also have added sodium and carbohydrates, which also increase fluid uptake from the intestines into the bloodstream.

Carbohydrate meals may be important as a post-exercise (physical) regime. If muscle glycogen is used up during exercise, it must be replaced. Carbohydrates assist in this process, and therefore should be eaten shortly *after* exercise, whereas protein should be eaten for energy before exercise. A better course of action is to prevent muscle glycogen depletion in the first place. One of the key factors in recovery and maintaining a high energy level is to produce more energy containing molecules referred to as ATP (adenosine triphosphate) and Creatine phosphate. ATP is generated by the oxidation of carbohydrates, fat and protein, and is used up in great quantities during exercise. It needs to be constantly replenished, and depends on the burning of fatty acids for this process. Creatine helps to maintain ATP levels.

Rhodiola rosea has been shown to increase muscle ATP and creatine levels, and increase the fatty acids in the blood. Adding Rhodiola rosea supplement *before* exercise, positively changes the protein balance in athletes and increase, the mass of contractile muscle fibers during workout. This results in a reduction in the duration of the recovery period. In experiments with 112 athletes, 89% of those receiving Rhodiola extract showed less fatigue after exercise, and improved performance in all levels of sports. The study confirmed a more rapid normalization of lactic and uric acid, resulting in less muscle stiffness and a quicker recovery from the stress of exercise .

STEP 5... THE CART BEFORE THE HORSE.

It's commendable to take supplements get yourself back to balance, but what about the gunk that has been sitting inside your body for years. Toxic colons, livers and even your brain can prevent nutrients from being absorbed.

We have to get rid of the manure pile. Yes, it may smell like that, because most likely the stuff in your intestines has fermented (bad food combining). I know few people who look forward to enemas and colonics, but sometimes they are the only way to blast yourself clean. If you would like a gentler approach, you can examine juice-fasting, psyllium seed, and herbal cleanses. Schedule these when you can get to a bathroom frequently and when you can afford a few days' sick-leave. Many times, the abundance of toxins being release from inside your body, may make you ill (colds, diarrhea, headaches).

JUICE FASTING AND HERBAL CLEANSES.

Juice fasting is not all that bad. At least you are "eating" something. You can either purchase veggie juices in the health food store (organic), or juice your own, if you happen to own a juicer-extractor. Blenders won't do. Carrot and beets mixed with greens and celery actually taste good to most people. Drinking vegetable juices separate from fruit juices is good food combining. Three or four days of this once a month is healthy for your digestive system, and will begin the detoxifying process.

Herbal cleanses are a little more vigorous. There are detoxing kits available that will guide you through this cleanse. Most times, they work through the blood and liver to draw toxins out, rather than act specifically as a colon cleanser. They can be combined with the juice fast. Some herbs that are used are red clover, hawthorn, alfalfa, nettles, sage, silica, echinacea, garlic, etc. An herbal detox tea may include birch leaves, parsley leaves and verbena leaves. Start with a three day program to see what happens.

Never continue cleansing fasts for extended periods (months and months) or you may have nothing left to cleanse. For liver cleansing, some herbs that are used in a body wrap, are ginger, dandelion root, capsicum, spearmint, bladderwrack and alfalfa.

Any blood and liver cleanse should dictate a colon cleanse, or many of the bad stuff will end up impacted at the other end. Enemas, colonics or an herbal laxative can help. Using psyllium seed hulls or powders can help by absorbing moisture and making stools easier to pass. Make sure that you drink lots and lots of water when you take psyllium.

Speaking of water, please make sure you drink only purified water, not chlorinated tap water or well water from high pesticide or nitrate farming areas. Bottled water is safer (depending on the consciousness of the bottler). Water treatment devices on your household plumbing are best. But, you must add back minerals to your water as the processing creates mostly dead water, devoid of life sustenance. When you drink this water, the body cries out for minerals and when it can't get them from the water, it starts pulling them out of your bones or other hiding places in the body. You become mineral deficient and are subject to all the illnesses thereof.

Combining a juice fast with an herbal cleanse is not only the way to health, but can safely help you drop unwanted pounds. This is a much better way to lose weight than fad diets, bulimia, or starving yourself. You are providing the body with proper nutrition while dieting. To quote Richard Simmons, "never say diet". This is not a diet, but an opportunity to give your body a nutritional boost. Obviously you can't eat the bad stuff on this cleanse. Therefore you will slowly lose your appetite for sweets (the real bad guys). Ten days without any, <u>and we mean any</u> sugar, will break the addiction and you will have less trouble with physical cravings, (mental cravings are another story). By just eliminating sugar and wheat (a common allergenic food) from your diet, you will probably not have to worry about gaining weight.

OUR EASY FORMULA FOR HIGH-PERFORMANCE.

★Start with a fast or cleanse, then...
★Take your urine pH every morning
★Take crystalloid electrolyte supplements
★Determine which acid or alkaline foods you need to re-balance yourself
★Eat high protein breakfast or whey powder drink
★Consume sea vegetables (supplements if you prefer)
★Eat properly combined foods
★Take supplemental enzymes with cooked or processed foods
★Drink lots of water between meals
★Maintain an omega-3/omega-6 balance (EFAs)
★Take a toddy of greens & nutritional yeast
★Add supplemental antioxidants and probiotics
★Add vitamins or other nutrients as needed

Additional supplements for sports training programs:
• bioflavonoids
• vitamin C
• Rhodiola rosea
• Rhododendron caucasicum
• calcium/magnesium
• herbs - gingko biloba, damiana, tribulus terrestris, mucuna pruriens, ginseng, licorice, maca,
• velvet antler
• HGH
• bee pollen
• B complex
• Tachyonized water

Typical menu for those days in which you will participate in a high-performance event.

Crystalloid electrolyte mineral water <u>upon rising</u>

Before breakfast:
Supplements in or with juice or water: nutritional yeast, lecithin, flax, neurotransmitter amino acid, Rhododendron caucasicum, sea vegetable or wheatgrass powder or caplet

Breakfast:
Protein food: eggs, turkey bacon, turkey sausage, whey drink, fermented soy powder drink
enzyme supplement

Morning snack:
(2 hrs. after breakfast):
Flax bar and water or
fruit and juice or
sugar-free cereal adding flax and lecithin with rice milk or wheat or barley grass juice

Crystalloid electrolyte mineral water
(20 minutes before lunch)

Lunch:
(1 hour after snack):
Salad, chicken or fish (not fried),
non-starch vegetables, sea vegetables
(no bread)
water, vegetable juice or herbal tea
enzyme supplement

Afternoon snack:
(2 hrs. after lunch):
One of: flax bar, avocado, cheese (no crackers), yogurt, nuts, apple
enzyme supplement

Just before event:

Drink mineral water. Take Rhodiola rosea supplement, green drink and eat flax bar or energy bar without sugar. No sugar, caffeine, soda pop, salty foods, carbohydrates.

Crystalloid mineral water
(20 minutes before dinner)

Dinner:

Salad, non-starch vegetables
choice of meat, chicken, fowl, OR
pasta, bread, starch vegetables and salad
Drink: water, vegetable juice or tea
enzyme supplement

If you want a sweet dessert, wait for 2-3 hours after the meal. If you want another successful high-performance day tomorrow, avoid sugary desserts, alcohol or caffeine.

Crystalloid electrolyte mineral water
(before retiring)

This menu is for those times when you need an energy boost. On other days, you may choose your menu based on the information presented in the earlier chapters of this book. Food combining is essential. A wise program to follow is one that includes an acid/alkaline choice of foods depending on your body condition.

Preventive medicine includes all the things we have spoken about so far. Since man is not perfect, some invader may take over and your body may need some help. If you have a specific problem we have developed a little cheat-sheet for you to review.

STEP 6... FIXES FOR PROBLEMS.

<u>(SYMPTOM: Nutrients to take)</u>

ANXIETY: Flower remedies - aspen, mimulus, blackberry, cherry plum, red chestnut, rock rose, Tachyonized water, homeopathic Gelsemium, bee pollen, herbs - skullcap, kava kava, camu-camu, melissa, (avoid stimulants like caffeine, sugar, alcohol).

ARTHRITIS: crystalloid electrolyte minerals, Plant enzymes, vegetable juice (cucumber, cabbage, black cherry) calcium balanced with magnesium, aged garlic extract, seaweed, spirulina, algae, nutritional yeast, EFAs and especially Borage oil (topically as well), royal jelly (from bees), herbs - nettles, red clover, yucca, burdock, cayenne, devil's claw, white willow bark, uno de gato, ginkgo biloba, vitamins E & C, niacinamide, zinc, velvet antler.

CANCER: crystalloid electrolyte minerals, digestive enzymes, vegetable juice (carrot, celery, lettuce, clover), aged garlic extract, EFAs (avoid heat extract oils), Chlorella, cereal grass, rutin, selenium, nutritional yeast, S.O.D. (antioxidant enzymes), Essiac tea, herbs - echinacea, chapparal, red clover, Rhododendron caucasicum, Rhodiola rosea, vitamins C, E, A, wheatgrass, Tachyonized water

ENERGY BOOST: crystalloid electrolyte minerals, wheat and barley grass, flower remedies, flax, nutritional yeast, chlorophyll, herbs - Rhodiola rosea, ginseng, gingko biloba, damiana, tribulus terrestris, mucuna pruriens, ashwaganda, maca, velvet antler, Tachyonized water, Human Growth Hormone, licorice, bee pollen, B-complex, sea vegetables, enzymes, calcium/magnesium.

EYE TROUBLE: crystalloid electrolyte minerals, vegetable juice (carrot, parsley, cabbage, kale, spinach, tomato), EFAs, zinc (for night vision), herbs - cayenne (for circulation), bilberry (not for Glaucoma), eyebright, bayberry, vitamin A (fish liver oil), Riboflavin (for cataracts), lutein, lecithin, bioflavonoids, amino acids, oxygen.

HEART DISEASE: crystalloid electrolyte minerals, enzymes, vegetable juice (carrot, beet), calcium/magnesium, chromium (with niacin), aged garlic extract, Chlorella, cayenne pepper, nutritional yeast, lecithin, EFAs, (no hydrogenated oils, refined flour, sugar, fried foods, meat, caffeine, alcohol), vitamins E,C,B_6, Thiamine, Rhododendron caucasicum, Rhodiola rosea.

HORMONAL IMBALANCE: (women-PMS, etc.): crystalloid electrolyte minerals, flax, natural progesterone (wild yam with progesterone USP), homeopathic (Lachesis), flower remedies, herbs - (tea from sage, Lady's mantle and horsetail) dong quai, maca, ginseng, black cohosh, hawthorn, chaste berry, licorice root, Human Growth Hormone, vitamins E with C, A (fish liver oil), flower remedies.

MALE IMPOTENCE: crystalloid mineral electrolytes, bioflavonoids, zinc, lecithin, homeopathic remedies, herbs - yohimbe bark, muira puma, catuaba, Rhodiola rosea, ginseng, gingko biloba, velvet antler, horny goat weed, avena sativa, maca, Human Growth Hormone, flower remedies.

MEMORY LOSS: crystalloid electrolyte minerals, aged garlic extract, lecithin, bee pollen, PS (phosphatidyl serine), herbs - gotu kola, gingko biloba, vitamin B6, (avoid aluminum and other heavy metals), flax, Neurotransmitter amino acid supplement with L-glutamine, DL-phenylalanine, Rhodiola rosea.

MENTAL ACUITY: sea vegetables, crystalloid electrolyte minerals, flax, wheatgrass, lecithin, nutritional yeast, phosphorus, bioflavonoids, Co-Q10, B complex, herbs such as gingko biloba, camu-camu, maca, ginseng, homeopathic Human Growth Hormone, calcium, magnesium, neurotransmitter amino acid supplement containing L-glutamine, DL-phenylalanine, Rhodiola rosea, flower remedies.

MUSCLE PAIN, SPRAINS, TORN LIGAMENTS: nutritional yeast, wheat and barley grass, crystalloid electrolyte minerals, MSM, calcium/magnesium, bioflavonoids, vitamin C, amino acids, ginseng, bromelain enzymes, aloe (external), Co-Q10, DLPA, flower remedies, homeopathic: arnica, hypericum, rhus tox, ruta graveolens, Tachyonized gel.

OSTEOPOROSIS: crystalloid electrolyte minerals, enzymes, calcium/magnesium, silica, natural progesterone (processed wild yam), bee pollen, royal jelly, herbs - wild oats, nettles, marshmallow root, yellowdock, horsetail (silica), velvet antler, vitamins C & D, Human Growth Hormone.

PROSTATE PROBLEMS: crystalloid electrolyte minerals, vegetable juices (carrot, turnip, orange, grapefruit, grape), lycopenes, EFAs, Chlorella, cereal grass, selenium, zinc, herbs - saw palmetto, thuja leaf, pau d-arco, burdock, uva ursi, buchu, juniper berry, marshmallow, velvet antler, vitamins C & E. (avoid dairy, caffeine, beer, pesticides, solvents, saturated fat, drugs, tobacco), natural progesterone.

SEXUAL LOSS OF LIBIDO: Women - fermented soy, EFAs, crystalloid electrolyte minerals, sea vegetables, iron, natural progesterone cream, velvet antler, flower remedies, herbs - maca, avena sativa, damiana, chaste tree berry. Men - crystalloid electrolyte minerals, sea vegetables, zinc, mucuna pruriens herb, natural progesterone cream, ginseng, maca, avena sativa.

STRESS: potassium, lecithin, calcium/magnesium, pantothenic acid, flower remedies, zinc, B vitamins, amino acid supplement, aged garlic extract, neurotransmitter amino acids including

L-glutamine and DL-phenylalanine, sea vegetables, herbs- hops, passion flower, suma, astragalus, uno de gato, skullcap. ginseng, valerian, kava kava, St. John's wort, ashwagandha, maca, camu-camu, shark liver oil, Rhodiola rosea, aromatherapy - lavender and ylang ylang oil, flower remedies.

RESOURCE DIRECTORY
(Who makes products for high performance.)

TACHYONIZED WATER™. Proven to be a valuable ingredient for maintaining radiant health, high energy and addressing imbalanced conditions, these drops, taken sublingually breaks the blood-brain barrier and instantly provides life force energy to the body. *Tachyonized™ Silica Gel* can strengthen skin, hair, bones, nails, ligaments and tendons. *Tachyonized™ Fizz-C* provides the body with 2 gm. Vitamin C and 7 minerals, all Tachyonized to magnify and accelerate their effects on the body's absorption and energy utilization. *Passion Dew™* is an extremely effective personal lubricant that will enhance your lovemaking and is water soluble. ADVANCED TACHYON TECHNOLOGIES, 480 Tesconi Circle, Santa Rosa, CA 95401 (800) 966-9341 Email: tachyon@tachyon-energy.com   www.tachyon-energy.com

PROGESTERONE HORMONE THERAPY. Useful in relieving the symptoms of menopause and lessen PMS. Remedies osteoporosis (renews bone density), helps prevent heart disease and protects against ovarian, breast and endometrial cancer. Corrects mood swings, migraines, vaginal dryness and enhances sex drive. Natural progesterone (derived from wild Mexican yam) is a safe effective natural alternative to conventional HRT drug therapy. *ProgestaPlus™* naturally restores critically important hormonal balance to help a woman regain her vitality, inner strength and youthful beauty. *ProgestaPlus™'* unique sealed pump dispenser delivers a fresh and correct dosage. AARISSE HEALTH CARE PRODUCTS, P.O. Box 210, Oakland, NJ 07436
(800) 675-9329 Email:jeff@aarisse.com   www.aarise.com

HORMONE HOME TESTS. Hormones such as estrogen and progesterone are fat loving steroids and circulate in the blood on fat-soluble red blood cell membranes. Fats and water don't mix, therefore blood tests don't accurately depict correct hormone levels. Saliva presents hormones at the cellular level where it is biologically active and can be measured accurately. Many women with high estrogen levels test low in blood tests, yet accurately high with saliva tests. *Evalu8™ Hormone Test Kits* are available for personal use. Hormones that can be tested are Estradiol, Estriol, Progesterone, Testosterone, DHEA, Cortisol and Androstenedione. AARISSE HEALTH CARE PRODUCTS, P.O. Box 210, Oakland, NJ 07436 (800) 675-9329

CHLOROPHYLL PRODUCTS: *DeSouza's Liquid Chlorophyll* is a versatile product that can be taken as a dietary supplement or used as a mouthwash and breath freshener. It contains no preservatives or flavorings and comes in capsules or tablets. The newly formulated *TOOTH GEL,* is a breakthrough homeopathic dental care product that includes baking soda for whiter cleaner teeth and potentized Cats Claw that is known for its positive effects on the gums. *TOOTH GEL* is free from sodium lauryl sulfate and contains legendary alfalfa-derived sodium copper chlorophyllin, an excellent breath freshener. Also available is *DeSouza's ORAL RINSE and SPRAY*, an excellent cleansing agent, astringent and breath freshener with natural cinnamon flavor. Only the purest of water is used, with Ascorbic Acid added as a preservative and it is alcohol free. *DeSouza's HAND and BODY LOTION* now contains Vitamin C which cleanses moisturizes and beautifies the skin. With this fragrance-free reformulated product, both men and women will enjoy healthy, youthful looking skin. DeSOUZA INTERNATIONAL, INC., PO Box 395, Beaumont, CA 92223 (800) 373-5171

www.desouzas.com

HOMEOPATHIC GROWTH HORMONE. *Hormonegentic*™ hand succussed homeopathic Growth Hormone (GH) 2C/30C. After age 25-30, levels of GH decline and that is when general aging signs appear. Clinical studies show men and women benefit with increased stamina, energy, strength, reduced wrinkles and fat, increase of lean tissue and toned muscle mass, improved eyesight, etc. *Hormonegentic*™ is the highest quality homeopathic GH available. Homeopathics are safe, gentle and free of side effects. DREAMOUS CORP USA, 12016 Wilshire Blvd, #8, Los Angeles, CA 90025 (800) 251-7543

www.dreamous.com

RHODIOLA ROSEA FOR ENERGY AND SEXUAL STIMULATION. Rhodiola Rosea, known for its energy enhancement, sexual stimulation and adaptogenic properties is our premier ingredient in *Essence Vital*™. *Forever Young*™ is the most complete antioxidant available at an affordable price, replacing several bottles into just 2 tablets each day. *Q-Gel Essentials*™ provide cost effective bioavailable coenzyme Q10. These and other fine quality products are available at FemEssentials, Inc., 934, University Dr., Suite 141, Coral Springs, FL 33071. (888) 866-6328 E-mail:jkycek@aol.com

www.femessentials.com

PLANT BASED DIGESTIVE ENZYMES. As Dr. Howell explained more than 60 years ago, enzymes are the sparks of life. *Genuine N-Zimes*™ is a full line of plant-based digestive enzyme supplements, including Dr. Howell's original broad spectrum formula. Other *Genuine N-Zimes*™ products include an extra-strength broad spectrum formula, condition specific formulas and enzyme activated herbals. All *Genuine N-Zimes*™ formulas increase the digestion of food, thus increasing the absorption of nutrients. All *Genuine N-Zimes*™ products are standardized and backed by decades of quality manufacturing processes. GENUINE N-ZIMES, 8500 NW River Park Drive, Parkville, MO 64152 (800) 929-7351

HORNY GOAT WEED FORMULA. All natural herbal alternative to prescription drugs. *Horny Goat Weed Formula*™ is a unique and extremely potent blend of herbs, specially coated to stop stomach acid from destroying their nutrients. This formula includes Mucuna Pruriens Extract (20% L-Dopa), Muira Puama Extract, Tribulus Terrestris Extract and Horny Goat Weed. These potent individual herbs have been used by healers to enhance performance, promote endurance, restore desire and powerful urges, and increase erectile ability. For women that have had hysterectomies, the benefits are similar. Also available, *TRIPLE STRENGTH GROWTH HORMONE*™, an all natural Ayurvedic herbal formula. This special synergistic blend of herbal extracts combined with a unique delivery system, produces a very potent and extremely effective growth hormone enhancer. *Libido Lift*™ formula also available. FOUNTAIN OF YOUTH, TECHNOLOGIES, INC., P.O. Box 608, Millersport, OH 43046 (800) 939-4296

NATURAL PROGESTERONE FOR MEN & WOMEN. Kokoro™, LLC natural progesterone cremes are on the recommended lists of nationally recognized authors. Natural progesterone is being used by women worldwide to assist with estrogen dominance health issues such as PMS, breast and uterine fibroids, infertility, early miscarriage, endometriosis, migraines, loss of sex drive and menopausal symptoms such as hot flashes, vaginal dryness and osteoporosis. A two ounce jar of *Women's Balance Creme* contains 1,020 mg (21 mg per ¼ tsp.) of natural progesterone. Men are learning how natural progesterone can aid symptoms of BPH, swollen prostate and loss of sex drive. *Kokoro*™ *Men's Creme* contains 396 mg of natural progesterone per two ounces (8 mg. per ¼ tsp.). KOKORO, LLC, P.O. Box 597, Tustin, CA 92781 (800) 599-9412 (714) 836-7749 Fax (714) 836-7476
website: www.kokorohealth.com

FRESH FROM THE FARM. FLAX FOR YOUR IMMUNE SYSTEM. A whole food, *Dakota Flax Gold* is all natural edible fresh flax seed, is high in lignins. Ready to grind, just like your best coffee, it is low in cadmium and is better tasting than packaged flax products. Seeds must be ground for full nutritional value. Dakota Flax Gold is available with grinder. Flax, also available in capsule form as *Flaxeon Jet,* is a convenient way of getting beneficial essential fatty acids. HEINTZMAN FARMS, RR2 Box 265, Onaka SD 57466 (800) 333-5813 (send S.A.S.E. for sample)   Website: www.heintzmanfarms.com

VELVET ANTLER CAPSULES. Historically, Velvet antler has been used for more than 2000 years in several cultures around the world. Since *velvet antler* is said to build up the body's natural resources, many consider it one of the most versatile all around health food supplements, and is becoming known as nature's perfect food. During antler growth high levels of natural hormones are present in the blood, including IGF-I and II which plays an important role in growth and development. *Velvet antler* is used to increase physical endurance, sexual fitness, stimulation of the immune system, blood circulation, wound healing, energy and for treatment of osteo and rheumatoid arthritis. MEADOW CREEK ELK FARMS, 7860 Woodland Lane, West Bend, WI. 53090 (800) 547-8450 #01   website: www.elkantlers.com

pH TESTING PAPERS: *pH Hydrion* Papers test the acid/alkaline condition of your urine. With readings of 5.5 to 8.0, these strips can indicate balance in the body and determine which food to eat to rebalance your system. LONG LIFE CATALOG CO., P.O. Box 968., Nokomis, FL. 34274 (888) NATURE-1

ALTERNATIVES TO DRUGS FOR HIGH ENERGY. Herbs have been proven effective alternatives to drugs for many ailments. *Medicine Wheel Herbal Drops* offer a variety of products. *HIGH ENERGY* includes herbs that aid acute exhaustion by supplying nutrients to the brain, circulatory system and muscles. *MEMORY BOOSTER* provides nutrients to the brain, increasing circulation, cell regeneration and cranial nerve function. *MALE BOOSTER* supplies nutrients to prostate and male hormone glands, increasing endurance, strength and potency. Deva Flower® Remedies reach the emotions surrounding symptoms. *FATIGUE/EXHAUSTION* is used when you are tired, or lack vitality and strength. *STRESS/TENSION* eases headaches and clears mental strain and muscle tension.   NATURAL LABS CORP., P.O. Box 20037, Sedona, AZ 86341 (800) 233-0810 Email: Natlabs@sedona.net

LIQUID CRYSTALLOID MINERAL SUPPLEMENTS: *Trace-Lyte™* is a crystalloid (smallest form in nature) electrolyte formula that helps keep cells strong, balance pH, facilitate removal of toxins and provide the body's life force. If extra magnesium is required, *Cal-Lyte™* offers a 1:1 ratio of calcium/magnesium with boron to assist absorption. *Total-Lyte™* is a 70% protein cracked cell yeast supplement that has been shown to increase mental efficiency, improve concentration, nourish the brain and combat fatigue. *Leci-Lyte™*, a unique blend of lecithin and crystalloid electrolytes is one of nature's perfect brain foods, and helps to ward off the mental diseases of old age. Improve your digestive tract with *Flora-Lyte™* for better digestion and *Colon-Lyte™* for total natural elimination.. NATURE'S PATH, INC. PO Box 7862, Venice FL 34287-7862 (800) 326-5772, (941) 426-3375 Fax (941) 426-6871

ELECTROLYTE DRINK. *Aqua-Lyte™* is an electrolyte drink that has no sugar or artificial sweeteners, dyes or preservatives. It contains true ocean-derived crystallloid electrolyte minerals (not sprinkled on trace minerals with electrolyte properties), and is in a base of pure oxygenated water which helps to facilitate the body's ability to metabolize vitamins, minerals and other nutrients. The combination is unique and supplies a missing link. OCEAN-LYTE ENTERPRISES, P.O. Box 531, Jenison, MI 49429-0531 (888)-NUTRITION

BRAIN FOOD FOR HIGH PERFORMANCE. As necessary ingredients for proper cellular neurotransmitter function in the brain and throughout the body, Omega-3 essential fatty acids must be balanced with Omega-6 essential fatty acids. Flax provides a good balance of these nutrients. *Fortified Flax* contains Organic Flax seed, Zinc, Vitamin B-6, C, E and is "yeast free". For a healthy snack, they also offer flax in a tasty *Omega Bar*, a convenient way to get your energy. *Fortified Flax* and *Power Pack Energy Drink* Mix can be sprinkled on cereal and sandwiches or mixed with juice or water. OMEGA-LIFE, INC., P.O. Box 208, Brookfield, WI 53008-0208 (800) EAT-FLAX (328-3529)

TAKE YOUR NUTRITION ALONG FOR THE WORKOUT. *Pines Wheat Grass* and *Barley Grass* tablets are a convenient and natural way to get nutrients your body needs. In addition to naturally occurring vitamins, minerals, amino acids, protein, enzymes and chlorophyll, Pines International's cereal grasses contain fiber which may aid in promoting regularity. After exercise, try *Mighty Greens*, a synergistic blend of superfoods, designed to provide high-quality nutrition and contains herbs which may assist in fatigue reduction. PINES INTERNATIONAL, INC., P.O. Box 1107, Lawrence, KS 66044 (800) 697-4637

ENZYMES FOR IMPROVING DIGESTION. The lack of enzymes in our cooked-food diets hamper proper digestion. This limits the nutrient absorption needed by our bodies to support our immune system. *TYME ZYME™*, an all natural <u>scientifically proven formula</u> contains all the necessary enzymes (Protease, Amylase, Lipase, Cellulase and Lactase) for better digestion throughout the intestinal tract. When taken with meals and/or supplements, *TYME ZYME™* <u>increases nutrient absorption by up to 71%</u> and assures the body of receiving the benefits of vital nutrients and essential fatty acids. This strengthens the immune system, aids in digestion, increases energy and improves mental alertness. PROZYME PRODUCTS, LTD., (800) 522-5537 call Debra Casey for information.

RHODODENDRON CAUCASICUM and RHODIOLA ROSEA HERB. The herb is consumed daily by one of the healthiest and longest living societies on earth - the people of the former Soviet Republic of Georgia. *Caucasicum™* contains the Rhodogen™ root of a rare plant grown at 7000 feet above sea level. This supplement also contains grain kefir containing 11 probiotics as well as the complex of minerals extracted from the Glacial Milk waters of the Caucacus Mountains. Containing lipase enzyme fat blockers, this herb is excellent for resisting body fat storage as well as being an excellent antioxidant. *Z-1*™ contains nutrients which support the body's natural cleansing actions and acts as a fat releaser necessary for effective weight loss programs. QUEST IV HEALTH/ Donna Faucher, representative (888) 217-7233

NEUROTRANSMITTER SUPPORT. *Restores*™ contains the specific nutrients the brain must have to *replenish* low levels of vital neurotransmitters, a key element in reducing stress and improving brain performance. Made up of a special synergistic natural formulation of amino acids, vitamins and minerals, *Restores* also promotes increased serotonin, dopamine and endorphin levels. QUEST IV HEALTH/ Donna Faucher, representative (888) 217-7233

INCREASE STAMINA AND PHYSICAL PERFORMANCE. 100% certified organic and Kosher wheat grass juice powder. *Sweet Wheat®* is pure green energy direct from nature. High in zinc and vitamin A, vital to a healthy prostate gland for men and necessary to promote a healthy hormonal balance in women. It contains live enzymes for better digestion. *Sweet Wheat* also helps skin and eyesight as well as fortifying the immune system. This formula enhanced with crystalloid electrolytes is available as *Electra Green.*
SWEET WHEAT, P.O. Box 187, Clearwater FL 33757-0187
(888) 227-9338   www.sweetwheat.com

MACA ROOT. *ROYAL MACA*™ grown in the Peruvian Andes without pesticides or chemical fertilizers, contains four alkaloids scientifically shown to modulate the pituitary. This causes the endocirine glands to produce a more adequate and balanced level of hormones, including estrogen, progesterone, testosterone, as well as adrenal, pituitary and thyroid hormones. It is effective within one week for hot flashes and vaginal dryness. Maca promotes mental clarity, a feeling of well being and sound sleep. It increases energy and libido in men (in less than 24 hours), and helps reverse impotency. WHOLE WORLD BOTANICALS, P.O. Box 322074, Ft. Washington Station, NY 10032 (888) 757-6026.

CAMU CAMU. *ROYAL CAMU*™ is the dehydrated pulp of the camu-camu bush which is native to the Amazon River basin. It contains more Vitamin C than any other botanical and has been shown to be an extremely effective antidepressant (works in a few hours without side effects). Camu-camu is also effective for anxiety and hyperactivity and is the most powerful botanical against the herpes virus in all of its forms. It resolves all kinds of headaches and has strong anti-oxidant and detoxifiying effects. WHOLE WORLD BOTANICALS, P.O. Box 322074, Ft. Washington Station, NY 10032 (888) 757-6026.

ALL NATURAL hGH PRECURSOR. *Unitropin*™ contains natural substances that have been shown in clinical studies to cause the pituitary gland to secrete human growth hormone (hGH). *Unitropin*™ is based on research revealed by Dr. Ronald Klatz, M.D., who states that amino acids and some B vitamins cause the pituitary to release hGH. *Unitropin*™ combines the scientifically proven benefits of hGH research, B vitamins, (including Niacin, B6 and B12), amino acids (including choline, L-Arginine, L-Ornithine, L-Tyrosine, DL-Methionine, Alpha Ketoglutarate and Melatonin) with co-enzyme Q-10 and crystalloid electrolytes. *Unitropin*™ also contains a powerful, unique life-enhancing blend of herbs and extracts is an excellent anti-aging formula for both men and women. Herbs for sexual enhancement include *Tribulus terrestris* (to increase libido, recovery time from sexual activity, strength of erections and increase self-confidence in both men and women); *Muira puama* (a powerful aphrodisiac, nerve stimulant and overall mood enhancer); and *Korean Ginseng and Ashwaganda* (that reduce stress and bring the body into a state of equilibrium.) These ingredients create a powerful "global" formula that effects both body and mind creating a synergistic sense of well being. UNIVERSAL NETWORK, INCORPORATED, 5647 Beneva Road, Sarasota, FL 34332 (800) 446-0302 Contact: Marc Pelletz   www.unitropin.com

RECOMMENDED READING:

Poisons in Your Body, Gary Null/Steven Null, Benedict Lust Publications
Make Your Juicer Your Drug Store, Dr. L. Newman, Arco Pub.
Acid and Alkaline, Herman Aihara, Oshawa Macrobiotic Foundation, Oroville, California.
Wheatgrass, Nature's Finest Medicine, Steve Meyerowitz, Sprout House Publications
Excitotoxins, The Taste That Kills, Russell Blaylock, M.D. Health Press, 1997

Books from ATN/Safe Goods Publishing
Order line: (888) NATURE-1

For a complete catalog of Safe Goods books call (888) NATURE-1 or look us up on the internet: www.animaltails.com

---

Crystalloid Electrolytes, Nina Anderson, Dr. Howard Peiper, $ 4.95

Curing Allergies with Visual Imagery, Dr. Wm. Mundy, $12.95

Feeling Younger with Homeopathic HGH. Dr. H.A. Davis., $ 4.95

Natural Solutions for Sexual Enhancement,
Nina Anderson, Dr. Howard Peiper, $ 9.95

The Secrets of Staying Young, $ 9.95
Nina Anderson, Dr. Howard Peiper.

Effective Stress and Natural Weight Management using Rhodiola rosea and Rhododendron caucasicum, Dr. Zakir Ramazanov and Dr. Maria del Mar Bernal Suarez $ 8.95

Self Care Anywhere, Gary Skole, Vivienne Matalon, M.D., Michael Gazsi, N.D., Bruce Berkowsky, Ph.D., N.D. $19.95

BIBLIOGRAPHY

-Aihara, Herman, *Acid and Alkaline*, George Oshawa Macrobiotic Foundation, 1986
-Anderson, Nina /Dr. Peiper, Howard, *The Secrets of Staying Young*, Safe Goods, 1999.
-Anderson, Dr. Richard, ND, NMD, *Cleanse & Purify Thyself*, R. Anderson, 1988
-Baldwin, James, M.D., *Cochineal extract*, Annals of Allergy, Asthma & Immunology, Nov., 1998
-Burke, Edmund R., Ph.D., *What to do when exercise is through.* Nutrition Science News, May 1999
-Christianson, Alan, N.D., *Ten for the road. Essential nutrients for endurance athletes*, Nutrition Science News, May 1999
-Coy, Chad, *Protein Powders: Whey to go.*, Health Products Business p. 34, May 1999
-DuBelle, Lee, *Proper Food Combining W.O.R.K.S.* Lee DuBelle, 1987
-Gittleman, Ann Louise, *Super Nutrition for Menopause*, Pocket Books, 1993
-Heigh, Dr. Gregory, *Shopping to Avoid Genetically Engineered Foods*, Sun-Coast Eco Report, April/May, 1999
-Howell, Dr.Edward, *Enzyme Nutrition*, Avery Publishing, 1985
-Jensen, Dr. Bernard, PhD, *Chlorella, Jewell of the Far East*, Bernard Jensen, 1992
- Lee, Lita, *Prostate Problems*, Earthletter, Winter, 1993
-Martlew, Gillian, N.D., *Electrolytes, The Spark of Life*, Nature's Publishing, 1994
-Meyerowitz, Steve, *Wheatgrass, Nature's Finest Medicine*, Sprout House, 1998
-Mindell, Dr. Earle, *Garlic, The Miracle Nutrient*, Keats Publishing, 1994
-Newman, Dr. L., *Make your Juicer your Drug Store.* Beneficial Books, 1970
-Null, Gary/ Null, Steven, *How to get rid of the Poisons in your Body*, Arco Publishing, 1997
-Ramazanov, Dr. Zakir and del mar Bernal Suarex,Dr. Maria, *Effective Stress and Natural Weight management using Rhodiola rosea and Rhododendron caucasicum.* Safe Goods Publishing, 1999
- Seibold, Ronald L., M.S. *Cereal Grass, What's In It For You!.* Wilderness Community Education Foundation, Inc., 1990
-*Understanding Vitamins and Minerals, The Prevention Total Health System®.* The editors of Prevention Magazine, Rodale Press, 1984

INDEX

A-C

acid/alkaline, 47, 56
alkaline, 56
allergen, 9, 26
amino acids, 28, 31, 32, 33, 35, 38, 39, 50, 51, 58, 59, 60
anemia, 19, 35, 37
antioxidants, 29, 30, 36, 45
anxiety, 31, 33, 37, 60
aphrodisiac, 39
arthritis, 5, 15, 21, 30, 37, 40, 56
athletes, 27, 29, 31, 37, 40, 41, 63
ATP, 21, 39, 41
BHT, 23
bone loss, 19
brain, 31, 57, 58, 59
Chlorella, 28, 49, 50, 63
Chlorophyll, 28, 54, 58
cholesterol, 32
coffee, 56
crystalloid, 57

D-E

dehydration, 57
depression, 14, 21, 31, 33, 34, 38
digestion, 9, 10, 14, 15, 21, 26, 55, 57, 59, 60
EFA's, 32
electrolytes, 29, 40, 50, 57, 60, 61
energy, 17, 21, 27, 28, 29, 32, 34, 35, 36, 37, 39, 41, 46, 47, 53, 54, 56, 58, 59, 60
enzyme, 61
enzymes, 9, 10, 11, 15, 17, 24, 33, 35, 39, 45, 49, 50, 51, 55, 57, 58, 59, 60
essential fatty acids, 20, 21, 25, 29, 34, 56, 58, 59
estrogen, 25, 28, 32, 34, 35, 38, 53, 55, 60
exercise, 3, 5, 10, 21, 27, 37, 38, 39, 40, 41, 58, 63

F-K

fast, 43, 44, 45
fat, 5, 11, 20, 21, 24, 27, 28, 29, 32, 34, 37, 38, 40, 41, 51, 53, 59
fatigue, 3, 14, 19, 21, 29, 31, 33, 38, 41, 57, 58
fiber, 58
flax, 56, 58
flower remedies, 49, 50, 51
food, 56, 59
food allergy, 10
ginseng, 39
headache, 3
herbs, 37, 39, 43, 45, 49, 50, 51, 55, 57, 58, 61
HGH, 34, 45, 62
homeopathic, 54
hormone, 30, 32, 33, 34, 35, 38, 39, 53, 55, 57, 60
immune, 9, 15, 20, 26, 27, 28, 29, 38, 40, 56, 59, 60
immune system, 9, 15, 20, 26, 27, 28, 29, 38, 40, 56, 59, 60
impotence, 19, 34
lecithin, 34, 35, 37, 46, 50, 51, 57
libido, 25, 32, 34, 35, 37, 38, 60, 61
liver, 34
low sperm count, 19

M-P

magnesium, 33
male hormone, 33
Melatonin, 61
memory, 3, 20, 21, 27, 31, 33, 37
mental, 4, 14, 23, 34, 35, 36, 37, 38, 40, 44, 57, 59, 60
minerals, 9, 19, 26, 30, 32, 33, 35, 36, 38, 39, 44, 49, 50, 51, 53, 58, 59
MSG, 23, 24
muscle, 3, 5, 11, 19, 27, 31, 33, 34, 38, 39, 40, 41, 57
muscle cramps, 19
neurotransmitter, 58
neurotransmitters, 31, 59

nutrients, 57, 58, 59
Olestra, 25, 26
osteoporosis, 33, 36, 39, 53, 55
oxygen, 35
pH, 17, 28, 45, 56, 57
pituitary, 60
PMS, 29, 34, 38, 50, 53, 55
probiotics, 14, 45, 59
progesterone, 33, 34, 35, 38, 39, 50, 51, 53, 55, 60
prostate, 38, 40, 56, 57, 60
protein, 9, 27, 28, 29, 33, 34, 38, 41, 45, 46, 57, 58

R-S

recovery rate, 21
Rhodiola rosea, 31, 33, 37, 38, 41, 45, 46, 49, 50, 51, 62, 63
Rhododendron caucasicum, 21, 30, 37, 45, 46, 49, 50, 62, 63
senility, 5, 19

sexual dysfunction, 3, 34, 36, 37
sexually, 32
soy, 12, 18, 26, 51
stamina, 27, 29, 33, 34, 37
stress, 9, 14, 30, 31, 38, 40, 59, 61
sugar, 12, 14, 17, 19, 21, 23, 24, 28, 29, 36, 38, 44, 46, 49, 50, 58

T-Z

Tachyon, 35
testosterone, 32, 33, 39
THI, 26
Velvet antler, 33, 39, 45, 49, 50, 51, 56
Viagra, 20
vitamin, 24, 28, 35, 36, 39, 45, 50, 51, 60
vitamins, 59, 60
water, 58
wheatgrass, 34, 46, 49, 50
xenobiotics, 35